How To Talk Dirty

157 Dirty Talk Examples Guaranteed
To Drive Your Lover Wild & Give You
Ultimate Pleasure & Excitement
Tonight

Natalie Robinson
Copyright© 2015 by Natalie Robinson

How To Talk Dirty

Copyright© 2015 Natalie Robinson

All Rights Reserved.
Warning: The unauthorized reproduction or distribution of this copyrighted work is illegal. No part of this book may be scanned, uploaded or distributed via internet or other means, electronic or print without the author's permission. Criminal copyright infringement without monetary gain is investigated by the FBI and is punishable by up to 5 years in federal prison and a fine of $250,000. (http://www.fbi.gov/ipr/). Please purchase only authorized electronic or print editions and do not participate in or encourage the electronic piracy of copyrighted material.

Publisher: Enlightened Publishing

ISBN-13: 978-1517509439

ISBN-10: 1517509432

Disclaimer

The Publisher has strived to be as accurate and complete as possible in the creation of this book. While all attempts have been made to verify information provided in this publication, the Publisher assumes no responsibility for errors, omissions, or contrary interpretation of the subject matter herein. Any perceived slights of specific persons, peoples, or organizations are unintentional.

This book is not intended for use as a source of legal, business, accounting or financial advice. All readers are advised to seek services of competent professionals in the legal, business, accounting, and finance fields.

The information in this book is not intended or implied to be a substitute for professional medical advice, diagnosis or treatment. All content contained in this book is for general information purposes only. Always consult your healthcare provider before carrying on any health program.

Table of Contents

Introduction 5

Chapter 1: A Brief History of Dirty Talking (Phrase 1-2) 9

    Why the Taboo? 11

Chapter 2: The "Anatomy" of the Dirty Talk (Phrases 3-12) 15

    Progressive Dirty Talking 18

Chapter 3: Your Motivation Behind Dirty Talking (Phrase 13-34) 23

    How Wordy Do You Have to Be? 27

    Flattery Adjectives 30

    Adverbs and Exclamations 32

Chapter 4: What a Man Wants (Phrase 35-50) 35

    Reprogramming Him 39

    Dominant Women 40

Chapter 5: What a Woman Wants (Phrase 51-61) 43

Role Playing with the Dominant Female. 47

Chapter 6: BDSM Kinks and Role Play Reversals (Phrase 62-70)............................. 51

Degrading Words.. 54

Chapter 7: Bisexuality and Taboo Fantasies in Dirty Talking (Phrase 71-78)...................... 59

Gay and Lesbian Experiences in Fantasy Sharing... 63

Chapter 8: How to Gauge What Your Partner Likes and Doesn't Like (Phrase 79-80) 67

Preparation.. 67

Putting Emotion Into It 70

Chapter 9: How to Feel What You Speak (Phrase 81-87)... 73

Concentrate on the Imagery 77

Chapter 10: 10 Dirty Talking Dos and Don'ts (Phrase 88-109).. 81

Chapter 11: Finding Your Unique Voice (Phrase 110-116)... 93

Changing Romantic Talk Into Something Kinky 95

Chapter 12: Free Sources of Dirty Inspiration (Phrase 117-129) 99

Lessons We Learn From Porn 99

Lessons We Learn From Erotica 101

Lessons We Learn from Phone Sex 103

Lessons We Learn from Cyber Sex......... 104

Chapter 13: How to Give Him or Her the Best "Sexting" Ever (Phrase 130-155) 109

Chapter 14: Dirty Talking for Every Situation in Life (Phrase 156-157) 117

Dirty Talk is Not Just Foreplay – It's Honest to Goodness Sex! 120

Conclusion 123

Introduction

Dirty talking—it's trendy, it's fashionable, and it's more acceptable now to get a little dirty than ever before. Maybe it's something it the water, maybe it's the newfound marketability of erotica and all the free porn that's opened our minds to pleasure, or maybe it's a cultural revolution. We're experiencing a resurgence of sexy thoughts, and women are just as excited to share their unfiltered fantasies as are men. It's the perfect time to be horny, to be open-minded and to be experimental. We have the toys, we have all sorts of encouragement, and we have nothing but time to kill titillating our imagination.

However, dirty talking is not as "easy" as people make it seem. There is an art and perhaps even a science to shocking the senses. It's not about what you say, or even the words you use.

And yes, there is a right way and wrong way to do it. As sexy as an all-night tryst might sound to you, if someone were to describe it **poorly**...

- *"Tonight we're gonna f**k and f**k. And f**k...and then uh...f**k some more!"*

- *"We're going to have sex all night. You and I. Umm...having lots of sex...sex all night, yeah, intercourse and penetration all night."*

The mood is gone, just like that! Actually, it's very easy to turn erotic and intense dialog into laughable stupidity. And just like the act of sex itself, if you don't know how to do it, you're just going to get the old "pat on the back" and reassurances of "We can still cuddle."

Don't risk killing the mood! Learn how to dirty talk, and do it right.

I can tell you right now dirty talking is NOT just a matter of:

- Using every swear word the sailors taught you

- Using every unsexy clinical term you've heard in rapid succession

- Overwriting your sentences as if you're trying to make your own *Fifty Shades of Whatever...*

Effectively dirty talking is a careful balancing act of expressing desire, of smart communication between two different lovers, and letting yourself feel the emotion of the moment. And yes, knowing your lover and what he or she wants is a big part of the puzzle.

So what I am going to teach you in this guide is how to talk dirty and how to do it right. We're going to learn what dirty talking is, the science of it, as well as the art of putting your own creative spin on the age-old hobby of talking your lover off.

I am also going to give you **157 examples of dirty talking** that you can use and analyze in case you want to improve upon them. That's the great thing about dirty talking in the privacy of your own home...you can borrow ideas all you want and adapt them to your own lovemaking habits.

We're also going to consider how you can improve your "craft" of dirty talking by taking in new information, practicing by yourself, and reading the signals of your lover. By the end of this book, you're going to feel like a rock star of dirty talking!

So let's not beat around the bush...er, poor choice of words. Let's get to the meat of the situation and figure out how to talk dirty...and hopefully without making any more sex puns!

Let's start by considering our long history of dirty talking as a species and our own Western and English culture. You might be surprised to learn that people thousands of years ago were just as filthy-minded as any Christian Grey or Jenna Jameson. As it turns out revolting against our sexual inhibitions is a battle as old as intelligent civilization.

Chapter 1: A Brief History of Dirty Talking (Phrase 1-2)

Sure, you probably remember a time when people didn't swear at all, less alone release their unchained sexual thoughts. You might think back to the Victorian Era, where speaking openly of sexual matters was considered course, and oversexed women were considered "hysterical."

Or perhaps you remember the golden age of Hollywood where nobody in the movies said a bad word and sex was only implied off screen. One of the most iconic movies was also the beginning of a new age in acceptable profanity. When Clark Gable said, "Frankly my dear..." in *Gone with the Wind*, it started an uproar.

People remember the Hayes Code of the 1950s that prevented indecency in movies, and how movies like *Who's Afraid of Virginia Woolf* forced the invention of a "Mature" label because of its bawdy and intimate marital talk.

However, few remember that well before the 1930s there was a sexual revolution going on in the roaring 20s, in stag films, and in blues recordings. Long before rap was assaulting our senses with F-words, our great grandparents may have been scandalized by Lucille Bogan and her plain-as-day sex lyrics that included these beauties:

> *"I got nipples on my titties, big as the end of my thumb;*
>
> *I got somethin' between my legs'll make a dead man come.*
>
> *Say I fucked all night, and all the night before baby;*
>
> *And I feel just like I wanna fuck some more."*

Thousands of years ago, in ancient India, horny men were pioneering sexual education in the illustrated Kama Sutra while China had its own awakening with Taoist Sexual Practices and I Ching. I Ching along with Tantrix sex, are credited with introducing the concept of divine sex, a much different Eastern take on sexuality than Western Culture, which through English Puritanism seemed to inhibit multiple generations with a fear of sex.

Books have always celebrated explicit sexuality. Long before there was *Fifty Shades of Grey*, there was James Joyce's *Ulysses* and Henry Miller's *Tropic of Cancer*, books that were banned for their indecency. However, they were centuries removed from one of the most prolific dirty talkers in all of literature, the Marquis de Sade, who was not only a self-professed expert on sexual matters (he was, oddly enough and ahead of his time for many of his concepts) but also thought to be a criminal because of his lustful appetites and explicit writings, such as in The 120 Days of Sodom.

Why the Taboo?

In the 20th and 21st century, it seems as if we are consistently going through periods of repression followed by great freedom. In the 1970s, *Don't Look Now* caused controversy for its explicit sex scenes while *Carnal Knowledge* raised eyebrows for its explicit sexual talk. The 1980s has *Fatal Attraction* and the 1990s had

Basic Instinct. Now we're experiencing a renaissance of uninhibited sexual imagination, where talk of threesomes, orgies and BDSM are the norm and penises are popping up everywhere, from movies to even M-rated video games.

Now is the time to embrace your sexual instincts. And that is the first lesson in learning how to talk dirty and mean it. Find your suppressed voice. Come to terms with the inhibition that has been forced upon you by civilized society and then learn to let go of it.

Because in dirty talking, there is no such thing as morality or as proper or honorable conversation. You're talking from instinct, you're talking from desire. You're releasing your lust upon your partner with nothing being held back. That's the turn on.

So even something simple like:

Dirty Talk #1: "I'm going to fuck you against the wall so hard...I want to see your face when you cum..." (Male)

Dirty Talk #2: "I'm want to ride your cock fast and hard...I want you to cum inside me..." (Female)

Is going to work like magic because it's the opposite of respectful dating conversation. Dirty talking is what everyone thinks early on in courtship, but what you can only say when you earn that special trust with your lover. When you earn it, let the fire rage on and speak what your heart...or more specifically your genitals...desires. Hold nothing back and enjoy the "shock" that comes from turning a good "friend" into a red hot love affair.

But there is more to the story than just rising above your basic instincts and screaming about fucking. There is an "Anatomy" to learn of dirty talking and it's not just about sex. It's about male and female roles. We'll discuss this in the next chapter.

Chapter 2: The "Anatomy" of the Dirty Talk (Phrases 3-12)

We know that to a great extent, the taboo of dirty talking is caused by social suppression and sexual fears. Why for a time, just the implication of the word "fuck" was deemed obscene. Not necessarily because of the spirit of how it was used; rather it was the etymology. Civilized and wealthy people used "honorable" language while savages had their own lower class way of talking. This even continued on as far as the 20th century, with "black music" and "black dancing" being perceived as overtly sexual and beneath white culture.

Even today there are clearly words we cannot use at work, in a press conference, amongst relatives, or around children. We don't say fuck, cock, pussy or cum in respectable company because they are perceived as intimate words. Words that lovers use together as a form of foreplay.

So yes, it is always preferable to use "four" and "five" letter words when dirty talking rather than speaking in a clinical context. "Intercourse" is not a sexy word. "Insertion" is not a sexy word. Even the word "vagina" and "vulva" sounds unnatural when talking dirty.

Erotic language tends to be short and clipped focusing on the heat of the moment and the obscenities we all know but never use in respectable, professional discussions.

Therefore, if you're a man your intent is clear...

Dirty Talk #3: "I'm going to rip off your dress and pound your pussy good. I'm going to pull your panties off and eat your cunt."

All he's saying in clinical terms is that he wants to take his girl's clothes off, have intercourse and engage in oral sex. In a clinical context, it's not sexy. But by mimicking the dialog of our own "lower class," which today might as well be porn stars, erotic writers, prostitutes, strippers and all-around perverts, we can turn a clinical act into something dirty. Something that would make another person blush. We turn our friend, our wife, our lovely partner who means the world to us...

Into our LOVER, our fuck buddy. Someone who's not deserving of "honorable" language and who we just want sex from. It can be your spouse, your best friend, or even your life partner from church. Because the language itself is not exploitative. You can swear at your partner all you want and still keep a relationship "clean" and moral. After all, we get dirty and then we wash. That tells you it's easy to maintain an honest and feel good relationship throughout the day and then turn into a dirty talking dynamo in the bedroom.

The female equivalent is similarly concerned with basic anatomy, taken from a clinical context and transformed into hot sexy talk.

Dirty Talk #4: "I want to pull that big cock out of your pants and suck it dry..."

Dirty Talk #5: "Fuck me with that hard dick...faster, faster! Shoot your cum all over me!"

Sounds a lot better than "Let's have oral sex!" Or "Shall we have sex tonight, darling?" doesn't it? Unlike men, dirty talking doesn't always come natural to a woman, since society has been extra hard on them over the years, suggesting that "respectable women" don't swear...even though have always gotten away with murder as regards sexual fantasies. This is slowly but surely changing during our sexual revolution and that's a great thing.

Women are realizing now that men do NOT look down on them for having a red hot imagination. They are not going to lose their "class" if they swear or enjoy phone sex. There is no reason for a woman to be prudish or "ladylike" and frankly that's not what a man wants at all. There is a time and place for everything and women can be just as filthy-minded as men. Keep conversation respectful outside in public...but show your partner you can be just as nasty as him when it's time to party.

"I'm going to finger that tight snatch...I'm going to taste your clit."

Progressive Dirty Talking

One thing to remember about effective dirty talking and "anatomy" of talking some off is that you have to "progress into it." As demonstrated, fuck, cum and pussy are perfectly acceptable to use. However, they might work best at the "end" of a sexual fantasy, just as excitement increases. Many lovers prefer to start slowly with sexy talk and then progress into the really filthy stuff.

For example, using a "finishing line" like:

Dirty Talk #6: "I want to pull your hair and fuck your cunt! Take it hard and deep! I'm going to fuck your brains out!"

Too early in foreplay might distract from the mood of the moment. If you're kissing your partner, necking them, or whispering to them, it might work better to take things slow and think of "softer" language to use at the start, describing what's happening. For example:

Dirty Talk #7: "Mmm...I love the way your skin feels against mine..."

Dirty Talk #8: "You like my hand on your crotch? Getting closer...and closer to your cock? It's so hard..."

You don't have to avoid the word "fuck" or "cock." You simply describe feelings and actions of the present. If a woman hasn't started oral sex yet, there's no reason for her to scream

"I want to suck your cock!" before she's set the right mood. As in whispering:

Dirty Talk #9: "Your dick is getting so hard. You like when I touch your cock?"

When she's ready, and things progress to the next stage, using a "harder" sentence will work wonders.

Dirty Talk #10: "Give me that cock. I want to suck it...I want to deepthroat that fucking cock and gag on it..."

So it's all about pacing yourself and talking dirty in "real time," not using the best stuff you have too early on.

Remember to think in terms of a sexual menu or timeline:

- The spark, the attraction
- Flirtation
- Making a move (Requesting permission)
- Kissing (Giving consent)
- Kissing

- Foreplay (Breasts, removing clothes, body massages)

- Prelude to Sex (oral sex, fingering, handjobs, etc.)

- Intercourse (slowly then progressing to harder and faster)

- Orgasm and Ejaculation

- Afterglow

Start planning out, vaguely, how your dirty talking progresses and take it according to the mood of the moment. You can also use tamer words at the start, such as "breasts" instead of "tits" or "penis" instead of "cock."

Something like this would be just fine:

Dirty Talk #11: "That's what you like...touching your breasts...putting my fingers through your bra...teasing your hard nipples..."

Dirty Talk #12: "Take off your pants...show me your penis...yeah I want to see it, baby..."

And eventually it would escalate into more explicit detail. There's no need to be shy...but then again, there's no need to "prove" how bad-ass you are by swearing too much at the beginning. Let's play it by ear and have some fun...just like real sex, plenty of foreplay is good!

There's a bit more to consider than just anatomy of our bodies. We know all about the cocks and pussies...now how about the anatomy of a sentence? Is there a certain way to write these X-rated sentences so that they sound less cheesy and more intense?

That's the subject of the next chapter...

Chapter 3: Your Motivation Behind Dirty Talking (Phrase 13-34)

Just as in acting, there's a certain level of "method" when it comes to creating sexy dialog. You're not just ad libbing this. You're entertaining. You're performing and putting on a great show for your partner. So take a little while to think about your motivation.

What do I mean by motivation? Think about what your partner wants to hear and what you want to give. Sex is a process of both giving and taking. Sure, you can be an excellent lover focused on helping your mate achieve orgasm. But at some point you want to feel pleasure just as you've given it. Therefore, in sexy talk, your intent is to:

- Say what you want to do to your partner (your desire to please, your giving)

- Say what you want to take from your partner (your basic instinct, your taking)

So yes, that's a safe "filter" to consider when thinking of sentences you should say and should not say.

Dirty Talk #13: "I want to eat your cunt out. I want to hear you orgasm while I look into your eyes, tasting your hot juices."

Dirty Talk #14: "I want you to suck my cock. Take that cum in your mouth. Lick it dry."

Both of these are an example of giving and taking, and are in line with what a woman wants to hear, depending on who's giving at the moment.

A woman's version might be:

Dirty Talk #15: "I'm going to lick your balls and lick up and down the shaft...then stuff that big cock down my throat..."

Dirty Talk #16: "Fuck me like you mean it...fill me up and let me feel that huge cock ramming against my wet pussy..."

Dirty Talk #17: "Lick my clit...taste my wet pussy and make me cum, baby..."

She's focused on giving and receiving pleasure.

On the other hand, saying something not related to giving and receiving pleasure sounds awkward and unsexy. Like:

- I want to bite you!

- We should have a threesome!

- I can't believe this is happening! Isn't this crazy?"

- Our sex life is so hot, isn't it?

- Are you enjoying our time together?

- Or worst of all, "How's your mom doing?"

Sure, there's always a time to ask questions like that, but it's not in the heat of the moment. Stay focused.

You might have noticed that the man and woman speaking these lines alternative between past tense, present tense and future tense. Sometimes they even speak in terms of what they "want," or what they're going to do. Just like writing and conversation, this is left up to your imagination. But it can help to think of the natural timeline progression of sex as regards description:

- I/You want...(what you desire)

- I am/You are...(describing the present; no need to say "I am" as this sounds formal, but phrase it as a question or a feeling)

- I'm going to.../ You're going to...(telling about what's going to happen)

- I did.../You did...(telling what just happened)

All of these can work and be mind-blowingly sexy, at any given time, provided there's a natural progression from start to finish.

Dirty Talk #18: "I want you to get undressed. I want to see you naked. I want your cock."

Dirty Talk #19: "You like the way I cream all over your cock, huh? Oh, you're fucking me so hard!"

Dirty Talk #20: "I'm going to squirt my pussy juice all over your face, how do you like that?"

Dirty Talk #21: "Oh God, you made me cum so hard. Your hot tongue made me so wet...I flooded our sheets!"

How Wordy Do You Have to Be?

In general, it's best to create naughty dialog in the same way you construct grammatically correct sentences. There is a noun, a direct object, a verb, and if you're really good, an adjective. So with a sentence like:

Dirty Talk #22: "Oh God...I want to suck your big cock so bad. I want to taste your cum, baby."

You have the subject (I), the direct object (your partner and your partner's body part), and a powerful action verb like SUCK and TASTE. You'll notice these are action verbs that involve one of our five senses. That makes the description more vivid and emotionally evocative.

As opposed to "I want you to be pleasuring me." Or "I want to be there, inside your pussy, pleasuring you." Sentences should not contain too many words, or passive words. Stick to emotion. To nouns, verbs and explicit actions.

And yes, it always helps if you can throw an adjective in there, because this helps paint more vivid imagery.

Dirty Talk #23: "I want to put my hands all over your ample bosom...I want to rub your taut nipples and pinch them, listening to your shaky voice crack and your tense body quiver..."

That's not a bad sentence, but it is the type of sentence that's easier to write than speak. You might get tongue tied if you try to say all that in one sentence. Or you might accidentally use a funny adjective and kill the mood. Reading erotic novels might actually be a little less sexy than you thought, if you get all sorts of bizarre literary descriptions for what should be a simple "Fuck", "Suck", "Grab" and so on.

For example, this is a somewhat over-the-top description with too many creative adjectives and weird metaphors. "I can't wait to fervently sample that delectable taste oozing out of your spunk-filled pistol like a volcano!"

Way too many adjectives and a rather strange set of images painted with inappropriate words. When in doubt SIMPLIFY! There's no need to complicate basic sentences with one dollar words. Sometimes the most obvious descriptive adjectives are the best. As in:

Dirty Talk #24: "Oh, your pussy is so tight! Yes, give it to me. I want to feel your wetness all over my cock!"

Dirty Talk #25: "Mmm yes, your cock is so hard, put it in me, fuck me...I love the feeling of your throbbing cock sliding up and down my lips!"

Nothing too complicated, just basic descriptions of what is happening and the feelings we have in the moment. And yes, you can get a little creative and come up with some great words to use, such as: throbbing, or erect, or bouncy, or whatever else comes to mind. Just try to keep your vocabulary common. If your partner has to think about what a word means, or about what poetic metaphor you're going for, it creates distraction.

Flattery Adjectives

You can never go wrong with flattering adjectives. In fact, it's a safe and effective alternative to trying to think up fancy words and descriptions. Just flatter the hell out of your partner with complimentary adjectives of their body and you can't miss.

Dirty Talk #26: "Oh put your thick cock inside my mouth! Face fuck me with that yummy cock!"

Dirty Talk #27: "Oh my God, I can't help myself. I just want to rip your shirt off and put my hot lips all over your amazing tits. I want to kiss every inch of that sexy belly."

Almost needless to say, but yeah let's say it...

Don't mention any "big" part of your lover that he or she might be self-conscious about. Big butts, big bellies, big hips are obviously a no-no. Some women are shy about the size of their large breasts or small breasts, so men might want to gauge how much they like "complimentary" dirty talking in this manner.

This is why a less descriptive adjective might work some of the time, such as:

> *"Put that delicious cock in my mouth..." (no mention of big, just to be safe)*
>
> *"I want to grab that sexy ass and smack it!" (sexy is always a safe word when you don't want to use, "big", "flat" or "bouncy")*

Of course, if you make your lover feel comfortable with his/her natural nude state, it shouldn't matter. If you show your lover that you like a "big ass" or in the case of a chubby man, a "strong" body, then the idea will carry through without incident.

You can also play it safe by describing emotional adjectives that speak about how you're feeling or your partner is feeling. For instance:

Dirty Talk #28: "Put your hot lips all over my swollen clit, baby..."

Dirty Talk #29: "You like the way I suck that nasty warm cum out of your aching dick?"

Dirty Talk #30: "My throbbing cock needs you...it's so rock hard it hurts! I have to fuck you right now!"

Dirty Talk #31: "Now ride my stiff cock with your hot wet pussy..."

As you can see, adjectives are usually not a problem. Say what comes natural rather than over thinking it.

Adverbs and Exclamations

Be careful about using too many adverbs or exclamatory descriptions. Using excessive adverbs or adjectives for that matter can be distracting. All your partner needs to know is that:

Dirty Talk #32: "I'm going to hungrily suck that big cock when I get home tonight..."

Dirty Talk #33: "I'm going to greedily eat that cunt until you scream for mercy."

These statements will work, provided you don't go into much more detail than that. "Hungrily" is a good word because it shows desire. "Greedily" also shows desire and lust. "Powerfully" might also work, since it paints an image and an emotion. Just don't get too carried away with irrelevant adjectives like "dramatically" or "fervently" or anything too poetic. If it comes natural to your vocabulary, you can try it, but forcing it out will only complicate matters. Dirty talking is not about being complicated!

Exclamation sentences and words, as well as intensifiers work to infuse the dirty talking with some emotion. You can't go wrong with old standbys like:

- "Oh God"
- "Jesus!"
- "Shit!"
- "Fuck!"
- "Goddammit!"
- "Motherfucker!"

And so on. However, avoid swearing incessantly for lack of a better word. There's no reason to say "I'm going to enjoy fucking pulverizing you all over that fucking bed. Suck my fucking dick." That's overkill.

But a more simple approach:

Dirty Talk #34: "I'm going to cum all over your fucking face!"

It works because it's in the heat of the moment and it's using just one intensifier for a climax. Simple is good, but repeating swear words too often loses the impact of a great "Fuck!" muttered at the right moment.

Now that you have a good understanding of "anatomy," both sentences and your partner's hot cock/pussy, it's time to focus a little bit more on the psychology of dirty talking, and more importantly, the roles you must play as a man or a woman. Let's move onto the next chapter and talk more about playing the part.

Chapter 4: What a Man Wants (Phrase 35-50)

You may find yourself stumbling occasionally if you're not sure what a man wants to hear from you. You may accidentally say something funny or too over the top, just trying to fit with the mood. That's fine and there's nothing wrong with saying something quirky and having a laugh. You can always go back to "sexy" within seconds. Practice makes perfect and the more often you dirty talk the better it can be.

That said, understanding a little bit about the psychology of a man will help you in coming up with the hottest dirty talk they've ever heard.

First, understand that a man desires to be attractive. He doesn't want pity from you, he wants to feel irresistible. Feeling his masculinity is what makes him hard. So don't be afraid to play the part of a wanton, lust-filled lover who is insatiable for every member of his body.

Dirty Talk #35: "You're making me so horny! Oh God you make me so hot for you. Oh fuck baby, you just know how to make me cum!"

Dirty Talk #36: "I love the way you fuck me doggy style. Hard and rough. It drives me wild!"

Dirty Talk #37: "I love the way you smell. I love the way you taste. I just want to drink you up..."

Dirty Talk #38: "Give me your everything. Cum in my mouth. Cum on my tits. Cum inside me."

In all these instances, what the woman is actually doing is flattering the man's ego. She's saying that she loves how he makes her feel, that she enjoys what he does, and that he has permission to do what feels good for him. Even when she tells him what to do, the message is flattery—that he can do anything and she'll enjoy it.

Traditionally, the woman enjoys being dominated by a man. Not all men will naturally play the part of a bold lover, so you may have to help the shy ones along, and let them feel like a take-charge kind of guy.

Sometimes reacting to their touches and actions is what they like best. Playing up your moans and groans, panting and squealing right when they enter you...these are all good ideas to butter up his ego.

Sometimes a simple stream of consciousness like:

Dirty Talk #39: "You're fucking me so deep with that huge cock, baby..."

Dirty Talk #40: "You like seeing your cock wrapped up in my big titties?"

Dirty Talk #41: "Oh you're making me so wet! I'm going to cum all over your cock!"

Works wonders because all the man really wants to hear is how he's doing a great job and how you want more of the same.

Sometimes flattery during sex is also a good idea:

Dirty Talk #42: "Your cock is so beautiful...you kiss me so nice...you lick me soooo good..."

This gives him the encouragement he needs to keep going and to intensify his efforts. It's also a great way "romantic" way to tell him what you want, rather than clinically instructing him.

Rather than saying "Now touch my clitoris here and put your mouth there..."

It's better to guide him along with your sexy sounds.

Dirty Talk #43: "Ohhhh shit! It feels sooo fucking good with you touch my clit right there..."

Dirty Talk #44: Holy fuck! YES! Eat my pussssssy! Eat my pussy just like that!"

Using exclamations works very well here, and eliminates a lot of the awkwardness of telling him exactly what you want. He will immediately sense what turns you on and respond to that.

Reprogramming Him

However, for most women there will come a time when their man goes in a different direction than she's comfortable with. This isn't always about anal or about fetishes, but sometimes it's just about what doesn't feel good to you. For instance, if you like clitoris stimulation but he's intent on finding the G-spot then it's not going to feel that great for you. He must be educated as to what you like.

The best way to reprogram him is to tell him what you like. You can do this by suggestion or by command. For instance:

Dirty Talk #45: "I love it when you suck my clit and lick it at the same time...it makes my blood boil!"

Dirty Talk #46: "Please squeeze my nipples. Just the thought of it makes me so horny..."

Dirty Talk #47: "Oh God yes I like that! Keep rubbing my clit just like thaaaat!"

In all of these situations you ARE telling him what to do. But by making it seem like you're getting horny it's flattering his ego. By saying, "try to do this..." you're offering a suggestion rather than a command. Not all men like being told what to do in bed; some find it intimidating. They feel they should be the master lover guiding you.

If your man seems to know what he wants, there's no sense in denying him that. Let him play with your breasts or look for the G-spot or whatever he wants. But after letting him take his pleasure, it's time set him back on course by pointing out what does feel good.

And believe this, once you start moaning and telling him what is making you orgasmic he WILL respond to it because he wants to send you over the edge. Making you orgasm is his mission!

Dominant Women

Many women will be making love to a less dominant lover, and there's nothing wrong with this. Not all men are naturally confident or dominant in bed, (even though the next chapter explains how you can improve in this if you're a man).

If the man enjoys you taking the lead then let him and indulge yourself, by telling him exactly what you want from him. Many men, particularly those raised in a suppressive environment discouraging sex, are attracted to older women (MILFs!) because they enjoy being dominated by a more seductive lover, rather than initiating themselves.

If this is the case then the dynamic might be slightly different.

Now a man wants to be seduced. As in:

Dirty Talk #48: "I said pull your cock out. There...that's not so bad, is it? Now I'm going to suck it...there, that feels good, doesn't it? See? I told you..."

Dirty Talk #49: "Fuck me harder. Fuck me like you mean it, motherfucker!"

Dirty Talk #50: You keep licking that clit. Don't stop. You use that tongue, little boy. You lick my cunt until I tell you to stop. Understand?"

In all of these quotes, it's clear what the shift in dynamic is: the woman is COMMANDING her man what to do. She likes it and he likes being dominated, or even "seduced" by the more aggressive lover.

This is the second part of the anatomy of dirty talking. The first part was expressing emotion and desire. The second part is commanding your lover and embracing the power you have.

Yes, men are usually supposed to be dominated in bed and most women respond more to men that are aggressive and more seductive. However, some men like dominant and commanding women. Some men are just "switchers" and enjoy playing both "top" and "bottom" at different times. One day he might want to be the bad boy seducer. Other days he wants to be the innocent kid corrupted by a temptress. Knowing how to play both roles is always useful.

Of course, if you are making love to your "alpha male" lover then he's probably not going to enjoy the dominant woman role. He might even find it intimidating or off-putting. If that's the case it's time to surrender yourself to his desires and let him take the lead. That's our next chapter. The role of the take-charge man.

Chapter 5: What a Woman Wants (Phrase 51-61)

A man who is naturally confident, or who at least is trying to play the role of alpha male, does not want a dominant woman but instead prefers a submissive woman who follows his lead. He wants to be the aggressor and the seducer. The woman doesn't start to feel pleasure until he wants her to. He is the "master" and she is the "submissive."

You don't have to be into kinky BDSM to understand the naturalness of these roles. Many women, oppressed sexually by a judgmental society, are more comfortable with men telling them what they want and then feeling the pleasure that comes from submitting to the dominant partner.

If you are a man and are not naturally confident then for the sake of role playing get in touch with your cold, macho and aggressive side. This is what most women want to see because a confident lover makes a shy lover feel more at ease. You remove the awkwardness and the "question" of whether sex is the right thing to do, and MAKE IT SO. You command. You give orders. You tell your lover when you to feel pleasure and when to give you pleasure. And guess what? She does. She responds to your commands right on cue, provided you mean them and follow up.

That's why using timeless classics like these lines work:

Dirty Talk #51: "Take off your clothes. I want to watch you strip for me. Bounce your tits for me. Spread your legs and show me your open pussy."

Dirty Talk #52: "I want you to look into my eyes while you suck my cock. Understand? Suck it harder. Use your hands to stroke it. Gag on that cock."

Dirty Talk #53: "You like it rough? I know you do. You lay back and you take every inch of that big cock. Don't you say a word. Your body is mine. Your pussy belongs to me."

In these quotes, you notice that all of the dominant male's statements are commands. He doesn't ask permission. His only questions are rhetorical. He doesn't bother asking for consent because it's assumed. He doesn't beg and he knows EXACTLY what he wants from her.

He also knows how to give her pleasure but instead of asking her how she likes it, he simply instructs her how to feel the pleasure he allows her. It's a role playing and it's not really politically correct or "feminist" at all, but it works. Because in the bedroom all rules are relaxed. You don't have to mind yourself so as long as you have an understanding.

You can still ask questions if you're unsure about how your submissive partner feels about a certain technique. (We'll cover more on this later) For now, just stick to non-permission based questions that establish your full control. Like:

Dirty Talk #54: "You like watching my cock go in and out of that pussy hole? Yeah I know you do."

Dirty Talk #55: "Are you a bad girl today? You want me to spank your naked ass? Like that, huh?"

Dirty Talk #56: "You sure like sucking on that big cock, don't you? Now take it out of your mouth and lick my balls. You like how that makes you gag? You like stuffing your mouth with cock?"

None of these questions actually need her response, but her yes responses only encourage him to talk dirtier, which makes her feel more aroused. Questions are just as powerful as statements, but are usually observational, mocking or even lecturing, as a Sexual Teacher. As in:

Dirty Talk #57: "Now you feel how big that makes my dick? Putting it in your mouth like that? Keep sucking on my cock head."

Dirty Talk #58: "Hold your big tits together while I fuck them. You like wrapping a big cock in those wet titties, huh? Is this what you were thinking about, huh? Me titfucking you when you first saw me?"

A teacher not only asks questions but gives the student an answer. Questions are actually used as "control" statements, making sure the student remains submissive. There is not really any permission expressed. It's assumed. And that's what makes it sexy.

Role Playing with the Dominant Female

If you're not naturally aggressive in sex, or if you simply like switching it up and letting the woman take control, then your statements will cease being as domineering. Instead, you will be helping the dominant woman achieve control and will be following her orders.

Your statements will be more along the lines of:

Dirty Talk #59: "Oh you're pussy tastes so good. Please let me stick my tongue in your cunt and lick you clean."

Dirty Talk #60: "Oh ma'am, please show me your nipples. Oh God, yes put your big tits in my face. You like the way I suck on them?"

Dirty Talk #61: "I just want to kiss you top to bottom. Put my lips all over your mouth, your breasts, your belly, your ass, your feet. I want to taste every morsel of your gorgeous body."

This dominated male lover does the exact opposite of the dominant. He seeks to please, asks questions and begs permission. He flatters her with compliments and she gives him commands. He responds happily to her demands and doesn't mind being lectured. Even his "commands" are soft, such as his request to "let me..."

Of course this dominated lover role play only works if the female assumes the position of Domme. If both lovers are shy and begging, the sex is still good, but it's not as psychologically intense as when one is seducing the other. The best sex results when one lover is in control and guiding the other lover towards pleasure—his and hers.

Now the next chapter is going to go into more detail regarding role play, and in particular BDSM and all that extra kinky stuff that makes for better sex. You will find that a lot of your "Dom" (dominant) and "sub" (submissive) ideas in power play can be expanded upon when you introduce these fetishistic elements.

Your aggressiveness can be heightened and your partner's response can be escalated into something freaky and well beyond that of normal sexual encounters. But this also gives you the opportunity to explore new types of love play, escalate your orgasms and fulfill some of your darkest fantasies.

Chapter 6: BDSM Kinks and Role Play Reversals (Phrase 62-70)

Really good dirty talk is always a little fetishistic. This is because fetishism is all about finding your "weak spot", what you find very sexy and taboo, and then focusing on it for heightened arousal and orgasm. BDSM stands for Bondage, Dominance, Sadism and Masochism. While much of what you see in erotic novels is considered "vanilla" BDSM, there's really no limits to how much fun you can have.

Most of that fun comes from the erotic dialog you and your partner create. Some couples are into role playing and assuming a different character in foreplay and in sex. Sometimes this works best because you or your partner might be too shy to actually say the things that you find erotic. So through the guise of a game or a role play, you can get away with saying something you would never tell your partner in real life.

For example if you don't like swearing in general then you might find it kinky to role play and say something totally out of character. Like:

Dirty Talk #62: "Oh baby, I want you to fuck my ass. Fill my hole up with that cock!"

This anal sex taboo topic might make your male partner really hot and it might make you just as hot. But that doesn't necessarily mean you have to actually try anal sex if you don't like it. Sometimes an erotic idea and a role play story is all you need to heighten your orgasm. You can talk about anal fucking while fingering each other or even through vaginal penetration. What counts is that you're both into it, not that you're doing it "by the book."

Sometimes swearing at your partner, as if you're having sex with someone you hate, is another dynamic worth trying. That's all part of the dichotomy of being the ideal spouse and the "mistress" or lover that satisfies your non-marital desires. Through role playing you can have both.

As in something like:

Dirty Talk #63: "You like fucking me, asshole? Just take what you want and then get the hell out of here!"

Dirty Talk #64: "Oh God, don't you dare cum in me. Oh God, I can't believe you're making me cum!"

This BDSM role play pretends as if you're coming against your wishes, as if you're being seduced. It's taboo but it creates an erotic sensation beyond that of typical sex. You're experimenting and having fun with the scenario. There really are no limits to what you can do.

The blackmail and non-consent scenario is very popular in non-vanilla BDSM, and role plays that you have special power over your lover. That you are the "master" and he/she the "slave." The slave doesn't want to do what the master says but has to obey, less the master become angry. For instance, the master could have a secret or could have strong manipulative powers over the slave.

Pretending to "resist" your master can lead to some extra horny and erotic dialog. Such as:

Dirty Talk #65: You may fuck my body...but that's all. You'll never have my heart!"

Dirty Talk #66: "Shut up and suck my cock! Or else I'll tell your secret and everyone will know."

In this role play, you can see that the man is clearly playing the "villain", and the woman the victim. It's straight out of an erotic novel, but it doesn't have to be that elaborate. Sometimes short stories of hot sex and "resisting" are all you need to have a glorious night of role playing.

Degrading Words

One of BDSM's most popular vanilla activities is using degrading words to describe your partner. This is not for all tastes, but some people enjoy the feeling of acting like a "whore" or a "slut." Prostitutes and strippers are common roles that women like to play since they are empowered, uninhibited and hard-edged. Once again, the opposite of the usual marital love that can get a bit boring after a while. These girls get paid to be fucked roughly and without love. And that's what the man may find attractive in an experimental role play since, of course, he's never going to cheat in real life. But the dynamic is intense and fun to try.

So if the man talks down to the woman as in:

Dirty Talk #67: "You're just a cum-guzzling slut. Do you want me to fuck you harder, you little whore?"

All the woman has to do is play "slave" and agree with the master's "discipline" and name calling. She may even take the lead if the man is too shy to "get into the role." As in:

Dirty Talk #68: Oh yeah baby! Call me a whore! Spank my ass and use me like your fuck-slave!"

If the male is playing the dominant he might not want the submissive to speak so much. However, if the woman is taking the lead and letting her man know it's okay to "act" then she might entice him by writing her own dialog.

And yes, you can easily reverse this scenario and have a powerful woman "ordering" around a young man to do what she says. Dominant female characters might be a teacher, a mother's best friend, a rich queen, a business woman and so on. She buys a gigolo for a night and orders him around, giving commands and telling him what to do.

A lot of guys will like this, as they still might have recurring fantasies of a powerful woman seducing them when they're young and vulnerable. If your man is not a natural charmer or "player", trust us, he will find the idea of a seductive older woman very hot.

Bondage is another fairly vanilla activity, though some couples do get very carried away with the whips, ropes and teasing toys! BDSM is not the main concern of this book, but yes, dirty talking can always be escalated using references to bondage and tying your lover up. As in:

Dirty Talk #69: "I'm going to take you home, tie you up and fuck you. You're going to squirm and try to escape but you'll be hogtied down. I'm going to fuck you until you beg for mercy."

Dirty Talk #70: "You like me riding that hard cock with your hands tied up, pretty boy? Huh? Now there's nothing you can do to get away. I'm going to make you cum inside of me. What do you think of that?"

Of course, these dialogs are not as powerful and arousing unless the other partner takes the cue and "resists" his or her captive. Pretending, for example, that a kidnapper or a crazy ex has tied them up and is going to sexually torture and tease them hours on end. It's an erotic story for sure, and if you can use handcuffs and ties you cuff your lover, by all means try it. What's great about BDSM dirty talking however is that you don't actually have to use bondage gear. You could even share your bondage fantasies over the phone if you'd like.

The point is, keep your mind open. Rather than shyly dismissing your partner's hottest and most forbidden fantasy, give it to him or her! Enjoy the role play and give yourself a memory that will last for a lifetime!

Speaking of taboo don't be surprised if your partner has an extra kinky fantasy involving another person. Read the next chapter if you dare!

Chapter 7: Bisexuality and Taboo Fantasies in Dirty Talking (Phrase 71-78)

It should come as no surprise to know that your lover, even your longtime faithful husband or wife, has thought about having sex with other people. Yes, it happens. And no, your partner is not going to talk about it or brag about it, because he/she knows in "real life" that's a definite no-no.

That's why the threesome or even foursome fantasy is so popular in dirty talking and fantasy fulfillment. We all have extramarital desires at times, when we meet an attractive new person, or perhaps have a friend we've always found attractive in the past. Surveys show that most faithful partners do think about forbidden fantasies a lot, and sometimes even during sex with you.

Yes, threesomes, foursomes, gangbangs, casual affairs, swinging, cuckolding, and sometimes even non-consensual kidnapping fantasies rank high on the list of fantasies we all have but never seem to talk about. So you have one of two choices: you can never discuss it and keep all those fantasies forever in the dark or you can have some fun with it and give your lover the gift of a taboo fantasy that drives him or her wild.

As we'll discuss a bit later, there is a proper way to introduce taboo fantasies and an improper way. But assuming your lover is into it, then go ahead and dive right into the surreal world of fantasy sharing.

You can act out the fantasies with role playing or you can even narrate a short story describing the taboo encounter. Deciding which "voice" to use will be a matter of taste, and you can also gauge how much your partner likes the idea by paying attention to the reactions.

The role playing game is simple. It would be dirty talking using a different character voice, perhaps someone you know, or if that's a bit too much for the green-eyed monster, then you can simply create a generic character similar to your lover's fantasy.

Dirty Talk #71: "Hey baby, it's me, your boss from work. Now whip out that cock and stroke it for me. I want to see you jack off. Don't tell me no or I'll fire you!"

In this example, the woman is assuming the role of the husband's real life boss. It's the same dirty talking routine but with a new flavor, since the image in his mind is now of his latest crush.

If that's a bit extreme (and granted, not everyone is going to be that all-embracing. Sometimes we really are too jealous to go there!), then a narrative format might work better. As in:

Dirty Talk #72: "You come and see what's waiting for you. I've brought you home a young stud who's nine inches long and hard as a rock. Don't you want to suck his young hard cock?"

It's not as threatening because it's not "about someone you know". It's just an erotic fantasy involving the man letting his wife pleasure someone else. It may never happen in real life at all, but in your dirty talking fantasy, you can create a vivid image and heighten orgasm x 10!

Instead of second person, as in "You feel this and you feel that", you can also describe your own fantasy and see if it turns on your lover. You could say:

Dirty Talk #73: "I invite my sexy girlfriend from college over. And we all get drunk. And then on a dare, she starts taking your pants off and stroking your hard dick. Then I take it and give you a blowjob. And then she joins it and we both lick your stiff shaft..."

Fantasies in the 1st person might work better if you want to "control" the fantasy and keep it within comfortable territory. Finally, third person narrative might work better if you're too shy to use "yourself" as a character in the fantasy. For example:

Dirty Talk #74: "Dave takes Karen to a swinger party. And they fuck in front of five other people. Then the other men join in and Karen takes two dicks, one in each hole, and the other in her mouth..."

Your partner may have different tastes, so it's fun to experiment.

Gay and Lesbian Experiences in Fantasy Sharing

This may be a challenge especially if you are not gay or lesbian and yet your partner is very insistent on having this hot threesome fantasy. Don't bluff. If you're not having fun it's not even worth it. Remember though that even if you're not comfortable touching and pleasuring a member of your own sex, there are ways to describe a threesome fantasy that are just as hot. For example:

Dirty Talk #75: "We take turns sucking your cock...I pass your dick to Amanda and she blows you while I lick your tight balls..."

Dirty Talk #76: "I rip your blouse off and present you as a gift to Frank, my new boss. He gets to do whatever he wants to you, that was our deal. So pulls your tits out of that hot pink bra and makes me watch. Him sucking on your titties is too much to bear so I start joining and eating your pussy out. Then Jake comes in and pulls his pants down. You suck him too, finally becoming the little gangbang slut you know you are..."

These are examples of male-male-female and female-female-male threesomes that are not gay, but still very kinky and may be hot enough for you to turn into a fantasy even if you can't give your partner a gay scenario. Sometimes just having sex in the presence of someone else, or letting them join in, can be enticing.

Sometimes foreplay with a same sex partner or incidental touching may be enough to turn your curious partner on. For instance:

Dirty Talk #77: "I take off Danielle's bra exposing her tits to you. Then I start rubbing her big nipples with oil, getting her tits all nice and wet for a double tittyfuck."

Dirty Talk #78: "My hot black friend with his ten inch cock is just dying to fuck your virgin ass. So I'm going to fuck your pussy and he's going to bend over and plug that asshole up. You like that? Feeling both of our dicks going in and out of you, just barely touching, which increases the friction...you're ready to cum so hard..."

Dirty talking is really a matter of negotiation and compromise. And who knows? Maybe you can summon up the nerve to give your partner a same sex fantasy. You never know if you like something until you try!

Thus far, we've reviewed a lot of ideas on how to spice things up and "turn up the volume." But dirty talking is not just about role-playing. Sometimes it's all about speaking what feels honest to you.

If you're feeling the fantasy, and not feeling the intensity of emotion, then a hot kinky fantasy means nothing.

It's time to learn how to communicate honestly and let your emotions flow in Chapters 8 and 9.

Chapter 8: How to Gauge What Your Partner Likes and Doesn't Like (Phrase 79-80)

Above all else, dirty talking is about communication, not just the taboo and outrageous. If there is a lack of communication, no kinky fantasy is going to make up for it. The heart, the mind and the true feeling of the moment is what makes dirty talking hot. You can read erotica all day long or watch porn, and still not be ready to give your lover a hot session of dirty talking. Maybe things are awkward or he/she just isn't feel the fantasy.

What gives?

Preparation

This is truly one of the most important lessons in dirty talking—communicating in advance of the actual dirty conversation. Don't ever "surprise" your lover with a non-consent or threesome fantasy, just assuming that your erotic voice and narrative will make him/her hot. You can't do that and that's only going to lead to tension. At best, your lover will "humor" you but not feel it. At worst, you may even start an unsexy fight!

Always discuss beforehand what your partner likes. You can talk about it in bed, right before the fantasy begins. Or you could talk about it in broad daylight, in a very logical sense with honest yes or no answers.

Since this is the "pre-interview" of dirty talking, you don't have to be romantic, kinky, or sexy. You just need information. All the kinky talk comes later once you learn what your partner wants. You need to know:

- What fantasies appeal to them
- What sexual foreplay and techniques they like
- What kind of person they find attractive
- What kind of setting they find arousing
- What dirty words they like

- What words they don't like (i.e. "slut is too much" or "asshole" is too much)

- What taboos are just right (i.e. "teacher-student is hot, anonymous sex)

- What sexual behavior is way over the line (i.e. no orgies, no prostate massage)

- What kind of person is OK to use for fantasies (i.e. no real life friends, no rape or toilet stories)

In fact it's best to discuss ALL of the above well in advance of even creating the fantasy. And don't be satisfied with just "I like everything..." Because that's not specific.

You ought to share with your partner your DOs and DON'Ts, what kind of kink you like, what you are curious about, and what you would NEVER do. This gives you the ammunition needed to create a titillating fantasy with all the right words.

If bringing this up seems awkward then agree to make a list of all types of sexual behavior that you can find through research. The both of you can check off what behavior is over the line and what isn't. This will help you negotiate a compromise that works for both of you. Sometimes the problem is not knowing what types of sex other people are having! Discussing it openly always helps.

Putting Emotion Into It

Putting real emotion into your dirty chat is paramount, because without it, sex—yes even that kinky thing you're thinking—is empty. No, we're not talking about love, we're talking about emotion and intensity. Sensation and excitement.

Are you putting yourself in the moment and "letting go" of your inhibition or are you still protecting and hiding? Your lover can sense it, believe it or not.

For example, consider two very different samples:

Dirty Talk #79: "Then we fuck on the beach. There are people around us but we don't care. All I want to do is grind against you, holding your hands firmly and whispering into your eat. I can feel myself inside of you, your pussy walls squeezing hard on my shaft and forcing me to cum..."

Dirty Talk #80: "Then I take you down on the floor, God, I just want to bury my mouth in those beautiful tits and smother myself. Pull your tits out. Let me see, oh God let me see. Yes, oh I got to suck them...let me suck them..."

Both of these lines are OK but the former is calm and centered, written for the female lover, and for her pleasure. The second example is grittier and more high-emotion, almost stream of consciousness and feeling the emotion of the encounter.

Ideally, you want to find a balance between telling your partner what you think they want to hear (which is not always fun for you) and also describing your own arousal and losing control. Your partner DOES want to see you hot and excited. So if you tell him or her a certain fantasy that doesn't turn you on personally, the emotion will be lacking in the story. On the other hand, if you're so excited about your own arousal and oblivious to her pleasure, it's going to be a one-sided fantasy.

The answer is easy. Get excited about the fantasy your partner wants to hear. You can take turns sharing one-sided fantasies, but eventually it's your turn to entertain your partner. You have to make the story about her (or him) and not just your own eroticism. Besides finding out your lover's secret taboo, there is a way to infuse the fantasy and dirty talk with genuine, uninhibited emotion. Even if it's all about your partner and not you.

That's the subject of our next chapter—committing to the fantasy and knowing how to turn ANYTHING into a hot and steamy good time.

Chapter 9: How to Feel What You Speak (Phrase 81-87)

First, understand that sexual excitement is always going to be male or female-centric. You can't really know what it's like to be a sexually aroused woman if you're a man, or an aroused man if you're a woman. You can guess but it's not the same as actually BEING the other sex.

So assume that what turns you on is probably reversed for your partner, since you're most likely two heterosexuals. We know that on average most men like visual stimulation, whereas women prefer emotional stimulation.

So if you're a woman feeding a fantasy to a man, expect that he likes it in that Hustler porn style, which is visual-centric, cynical and raw.

As in:

Dirty Talk #81: "Oh yeah, you want my big wet titties all over your cock? Is that what you've been thinking about? Lemme spit on it and get it all nice and wet so I can titfuck you. I'm going to wrap my tits around the shaft and then suck on the head. Just like you want it, pervert!"

Dirty Talk #82: "Oh my pussy lips are so soft squeezing your cockhead. My cum is dripping all over your cock...you're going to make me squirt all over you!"

And you notice she's emphasizing her own body parts, knowing that's what turns him on. She mentions his penis in passing but her breasts, vagina and lips are the key images that enthrall him.

Men have to adapt to the female-centric view of sex, emphasizing their body parts and how he interacts with her. Such as:

Dirty Talk #83: "Now take my cock inside you. Feel how hard my dick is? My throbbing cock slides in and out of you and you can feel every vein ribbing against your wall. My cockhead rubs against your sweet spot and you feel a shudder. My balls slap against your ass as I start thrusting harder and harder..."

Dirty Talk #84: I eat you out as you sit in your office chair, looking up at you, keeping hard eye contact. I want you to see my eyes, see my passion for you, while you spill onto me. Look at me when I make you cum. Look at my tongue teasing you. Yeah that's it, grab my hair and shove me deeper inside. I'm going tongue-fuck you until you scream..."

He's focusing his attention on his male parts, and his face, all of his body, as he interacts with his female partner. You might think it's self-centered to talk about your own body instead of your partners, but it's actually more attune with their natural instincts. Women know what parts they have. But they're fascinated by the penis. Men are fascinated by breasts and the vagina. This is what turns us on. So try thinking "in reverse" in terms of anatomy.

A lot of women also prefer a more literate and emotional prelude to hard dirty talk. Now we're not saying that women are embarrassed to get down and dirty, far from it. But setting up the scene before diving right into the vagina and breasts works brilliantly. For example:

Dirty Talk #85: "Imagine you're on a cruise ship. Alone and looking out at the sea. You're a bit tipsy after that wine. You're dancing to the music you still hear coming from the inside of the party room. Suddenly you feel a strong male presence behind you. A man's hand slips into the top of your backless halter and cups your breasts with his firm hands. You don't know who it is, but his hot breath and deep breathing are turning you on. As he begins groping your tits you realize you don't care. You just want to be fucked. He pulls one hand out so that he can finger you, right there, in public. You're too turned on to say no. You reach around and feel his bulging cock getting harder..."

Now in this fantasy dirty talk, you notice not only is that man emphasizing his own parts, but more important he's describing the MOOD of a scene. He's telling her how to feel, what she feels, rather than just telling her how hard he's fucking her. Her mood is captivated at the "story" and the attention to the environment. From that point on, he can say "fuck" and "tits" all he wants because he's already stimulated her emotions and involved her in the scene. And all it took to put her on slow boil was just taking a minute to set a mood without swearing.

Of course, it's not just a woman's thing. Believe this, if a woman takes the time to set up a scene and a mood, the man will be just as aroused and into it. The only real difference is that whereas a woman can imagine hot sex aboard a ship, a man's fantasy might usually delve deeper into outrageous scenarios. He doesn't need to be seduced...he's ready to go!

Concentrate on the Imagery

When you're dirty talking to each other, you use both visual and aural stimulation as well as words that evoke all five senses. You won't literally smell or taste anything, especially if you're talking on the phone or online. So it's best to paint strong visual images through language. Besides, even if you are having sex, you can do no wrong with spicy visuals thrown in at key parts.

Focus on:

- Sexual positions or foreplay
- Sights that he/she might see

- Expressions on his/her face
- The level of his or her excitement
- What he or she is feeling, and how arousal intensifies
- Details about penetration

Two examples would be:

Dirty Talk #86: "I pull my hard cock out and start rubbing it all over your hot and quivering pussy. I trace it down your pussy lips and then rub my head all over your clit. I make you watch, grabbing your hair, and making you watch as I shove my cock back in and thrust deeper..."

Dirty Talk #87: "I'm riding you so hard with my wet cunt I'm shaking the bed. All you can hear is the bed legs creaking back and forth...that is until I start screaming and squirting and not slowing down one bit. I'm going to grind on this cock until you explode! All you can smell is my pussy and that makes you crazy. You shoot ten spurts into me and I lean back giving you a full view of my neatly trimmed bush..."

Details, including the ones not directly related to penetration, (such as the sound the bed is making, or the smell of her lubricant) make all the difference!

By now you have a pretty good idea of how to get started dirty-talking. You know the anatomy and how to infuse your chat with lust, emotion, imagery and mood. However, you're not going to get it perfectly down pat the first few times. Don't let occasional mishaps embarrass you or discourage you from trying again.

What might help steer you back to the right course is knowing what to do and what to avoid. That's the subject of our next chapter.

Chapter 10: 10 Dirty Talking Dos and Don'ts (Phrase 88-109)

Remember these 10 commandments of dirty talking so you can avoid awkwardness, excessive laughter, or the dreaded dead bed syndrome. (Which is when your partner just gives up on you because you've failed so miserably) Stick to these tips and you should be fine:

DO 1: Use experiences from your normal life to zing up the chemistry. It puts your heart into it and gives you the energy to follow through with a new fantasy.

Dirty Talk #88: "Remember that girl who was hitting on you at the store? What if I invited her over for a threesome and we both took turns tonguing your cock?"

Dirty Talk #89: "Remember that time vacationing in Florida? We joked about having sex right there in public in front of all those people. I think we should it next time. Wouldn't you enjoy being watched while you ride me in the hot tub?"

Or something a little more gentle like:

Dirty Talk #90: "I saw you looking at those cheerleaders. Maybe I should dress up in a cheerleader's outfit and we can go behind the bleachers. Just like old times? Fucking like mad everywhere we went?"

Dirty Talk #91: "All this dressing up lately has got me horny. We should go down on each other in the bathroom while keeping our clothes on. See if we can do a quick fuck without anyone suspecting."

DO NOT: Be shy. Don't hold back. There's no sense in getting dirty and extreme if you're too shy to say what you feel. And don't react badly if your partner gets kinkier than you imagined. Be happy that he/she trusts you enough to confide. That doesn't mean you have to do "everything." Just make compromises as best you can so that both of you are happy.

DO 2: Always give feedback. Don't just sit there in awkward silence and don't just sit there and enjoy it. Give your partner encouragement because he/she is basing the next few lines of the fantasy chat on your honest reactions. You help tell the story, you fire up the imagination. The stuff you like react more. The stuff you're not crazy about react less.

Dirty Talk #92: "Oh God! (He speaks) Yeah I like that! (He asks a question) Yes, master. Please spank me again. (He talks about sex on the desk) Yes, fuck me right on my desk! Ooooh! (He asks a question) Yes yes yes yes! Don't ever stop fucking me!"

DO NOT: Interrupt, talk over or mock the other person. Try to avoid laughing if possible. It's like a dance. When one is leading the other follows. If you do laugh or say something unsexy by accident just continue on and don't dwell on it.

DO 3: Look into his/her eyes. Or if you're not together in person then describe looking into each other's eyes, or looking at each other's body and genitals. This is a strong visual and helps create bonding and intimacy, even through the power of suggestion.

Dirty Talk #93: "Look at me. I want you to orgasm looking into my eyes. I want to feel you quake on top of me and let go, giving me your whole body. Look at me...look at me while we cum together..."

DO NOT: Be demeaning or critical. Even if you and your partner is into name calling and BDSM humiliation, that's still better than being "helpfully" critical of your lover's performance. That is the absolute worst thing you can do, because you rob them of all confidence. Do not interrupt your partner to tell him/her what's wrong. Instead, use POSITIVE feedback and encouragement to reward good behavior.

DO 4: Always tell your partner that he or she is sexy. And don't just do it once, but reassure them throughout the whole session. This builds confidence. There are some BDSM activities that involve insulting your partner, but for the most part, this is not recommended for novices. Make him or her feel confident in their body, flaws and all.

Dirty Talk #94: "Oh God you're so sexy when you touch yourself and look at me. I love your body. You turn me on so much when look me in the eyes..."

DO NOT: Get too technical or too elaborate. This is usually what messes you up and tongue-ties you. Don't take too much time describing a strange sexual position or the various items around a room. Those are irrelevant details. A simple statement describing what's happening in one sentence is just fine, as in:

Dirty Talk #95: "I push you down on the desk and fuck you sideways, resting your leg on my shoulder while I enter you..."

DO 5: Use your partner's name. Even if it's a play name or a fictional character, calling someone's name and making the emotion more intimate, always has a profound effect.

Dirty Talk #96: "Oh Veronica...I want to make love to you like mad. Every time I think of your name, Veronica, the sound sends a shiver down my spine..."

DON'T: Feel pressured to have an orgasm or do things/say things that make you uncomfortable. The whole experience will be miserable if you force yourself to do anything. This is about no pressure, experimentation and having fun.

DO 6: Tell your lover how appealing they are to all senses. You know by now you have to compliment your lover's beauty. But don't stop there. Take time to comment on his/her smell, taste, their texture and skin, and their voice. Involving all five senses helps keeps things alive and intense.

Dirty Talk #97: "Mmm you taste so good I just want to lick you up like cool whip. Taste every crevice of your delicious body."

DON'T: Talk too much. You should talk frequently but don't get fixated on perfectly describing a scene or a certain maneuver. The images and the mood is what counts, not the word usage or the exact position. Stick to a number of short and progressive sentences rather than trying to keep telling the same sentence in a different way.

DO 7: Keep your lover updates about your level of arousal. Timing your orgasms close to each other is always a better idea than coming prematurely or taking too long. Rather than saying it matter-of-factly, tell them in a sexy way how you feel, and let it be clear what this means. For example:

Dirty Talk #98: "My pussy's getting so dripping wet hearing you talk like that..." (Entry is OK)

Dirty Talk #99: Oh you're going to make me cum soon... (almost to climax)

Dirty Talk #100: "Oh God, you're making me too horny...I want to turn you around and fuck you now...(This can be used as a sexy way of saying to change positions just in case the man is too close to coming)

DO 8: Ask more open-ended questions. While masters and doms usually ask rhetorical questions, you might need a little more encouragement this early on. Open-ended questions can help guide your lover to where you need to be for him/her to orgasm. Knowing that criticism is not a good thing, give your lover the opportunity to answer open-ended questions for better understanding, not just yes or no questions. For instance:

Dirty Talk #101: "Where do you like to be touched, slave?"

Dirty Talk #102: "Where are you most sensitive? Where am I forbidden to touch?"

Dirty Talk #103: "Tell me where you want to cum, lover. You can cum anywhere."

In these instances, notice that even when asking for information, the dominant lover didn't break the mood. He/she just asked where the submissive wanted to be touched, as if offering an option, but still controlled the session. No begging, no asking permission.

DON'T: Use physical characteristics that are simply not true. While "big cock" or "big tits" are nice for an erotic fantasy, if your partner has average size parts, then you're only going to sound insincere. Instead, try using neutral-size words like firm cock, luscious breasts, wet pussy, and so on.

DO 9: When in doubt, move slower. Dirty talking should be about slow-boil and about extending the moment into an all-nighter. Don't start off too rough, don't use too many sledgehammer vulgarities in the first five minutes. Work your way towards it. You could even spend a lot of time focusing on breast play and give her an orgasm before the really dirty stuff begins.

Dirty Talk #104: "I'm going to slide my fingers into your bra and touch your nipples. Slowly at first, gently tracing a circle with my finger. Then tap your erect nipple making it taunt. Then pinch it slightly, getting you aroused..." (Step by step until she's begging for more intensity)

DON'T: Don't repeat yourself. This may be challenging at times, especially if your lover is taking an unusually long time to orgasm. Don't pressure them and don't keep repeating the same sentences or rewriting them either. If you try to extend the fantasy longer than it should go, hoping to match your lover's timing of orgasm, you may get tongue-tied and run out of things to say. In general, this is why it's better to start slow and progress slowly rather than jumping into finishing climaxes. If you run out of sentences, then simply change the position of the fantasy, or concentrate on another part of her body. That way, you're changing the idea and the current, without losing the scene itself. Don't start a brand new scene, to avoid losing the mood you have so far.

Dirty Talk #105: "Did you like being fucked doggy style? Now turn over because I want to look at your face while I fuck you spread eagle. I want to see my cock go in deep..."

Dirty Talk #106: Now there's another mysterious stranger who walks up behind you. I tell him to fuck you too. We're all going to use you as our play toy. Get ready to quake and quake.

DO 10: Remember to focus on your tone: your pitch, power and pace in your voice. A sexually charged voice has moderately loud volume which increases when orgasm is imminent. You can also have a sexier voice my lowering your pitch and taking on a deeper, more mysterious and more lustful tone. Finally, if you're just getting started and feeling sensual then talk slower than average. As you become excited, your breathing increases and your words come out faster from your mouth. To some extent all of this is involuntary when you're aroused. But just in case you're talking too dryly or at an even temper, you can purposely exercise your vocal chords for a hotter experience.

Dirty Talk #107: "Let me touch you...right there...on your budding clit...notice how your back is arching in arousal. You want me...to keep touching you...don't you?" (Slowing down for a steamier introduction)

Dirty Talk #108: "I said take your clothes off. Today, you're going to do whatever I say." (A firm voice with slightly higher volume)

Dirty Talk #109: "Oh yes yes! More! Faster! God I love the way you lick my clit just like that ohh keep going keep going fuck me oh God make me cum! (Fast sentences that eventually become run on sentences as orgasm comes; the intensity of the sensation breaks down logical sentences to frantic exclamations of emotion)

DO NOT: Take chances by saying something you haven't agreed upon yet. Don't risk it, even if it's something you figure "everyone" is doing. That violates trust and WILL make things awkward for a long time to come.

Now that we understand a bit more about what to avoid and what to do, let's talk about making dirty talk "your own" by bringing your unique voice into the equation.

Chapter 11: Finding Your Unique Voice (Phrase 110-116)

So much of dirty talking comes from what we hear other people say, whether in movies, TV or books. And that might work for a time, especially if you're just starting out. However, as you improve your technique and gain practice in this wonderful "pastime", you will start to turn all your erotic "borrowed" ideas into your own unique pattern.

As you realize that yes, it really is YOU dirty talking and not Mr. Pornstar or Mr. Sexy Billionaire that is only going to fill you with self-confidence and turn your partner on. Sex and dirty talking is about the personal experience, the honest and unfiltered communication between two people who have found each other. This is a great connection of spirit, mind and soul and it's time to explore every inch and every idea in each other's company.

So remember:

- Be yourself. If something doesn't feel right when you say it, stop saying it. If a fantasy doesn't turn you on, just let it go and try something else. Sex is like a menu and you can have anything you want!

- Borrow your ideas from others but rewrite them in your own words. Don't use words you're not accustomed to. Instead, translate them into your own unique language – like something your partner can imagine you saying.

- Practice by yourself, whether aloud or silently. Practice makes perfect and you can work on your sex talking technique privately so you can impress your spouse next time with some vivid descriptions.

- Make sure your emotions are always invested. If it's your spouse's fantasy try to summon up your own feelings and focus on the details that turn you on. Don't just tell your partner what you think they want to hear—make yourself part of the fantasy and own the moment, losing your inhibitions just a little bit.

Changing Romantic Talk Into Something Kinky

One challenge for inexperienced dirty talkers is to turn their romantic feelings into something kinky and dirty. If you're not naturally profane and hardly ever swear in normal life, and are not into anything too kinky, dirty talking will not come naturally to you.

If this is the case it's time to "transform" some of your innocent observations about love into something a little more usable for the sake of your partner's fantasies. For example...

Innocent Remark:

"I love my partner with my whole heart."

Becomes:

Dirty Talk #110: "I want you so bad...I'll let you do ANYTHING to me. Anything!"

Innocent Remark:

"Every time I see you, you make me smile."

Becomes:

Dirty Talk #111: "I'm addicted to your cock/pussy. I want to taste you. I want to fuck you always. I NEED you now!"

Innocent Remark:

"I want to have a family with you."

Becomes:

Dirty Talk #112: "Give your hot jizz, baby. Fill me up with that baby maker and feed it all to me!"

Innocent Remark:

"I love your adorable smile."

Becomes:

Dirty Talk #113: "I want to look at your pretty face when you deepthroat my cock."

Dirty Talk #114: "Look at me. Don't you dare stop looking at me. Eat my pussy juices while you fuck me with those hungry eyes."

Innocent Remark:

"I feel so close to you right now."

Becomes:

Dirty Talk #115: "I want to feel you from the inside. I want our bodies and fluids to mesh together. I want your cum, sweat, tears and spit. I just want to drink you up."

Innocent Remark:

"We should go out to the park and have a romantic picnic."

Becomes:

Dirty Talk #116: "We should go to some isolated area. Eat, drink and then fuck like crazy teens behind the bushes."

As you can see, dirty thoughts are nothing more than compliments rewritten to be sexual. So learn to use your normal thoughts as fodder for making some truly graphic and X-rated conversation. We know you have a filthy mind! Everyone does...

Speaking of which, just how helpful are all these other outside sources like porn, erotica books, movies and the like? Let's find out in Chapter 12.

Chapter 12: Free Sources of Dirty Inspiration (Phrase 117-129)

If you're still feeling a bit shy about practicing your X-rated diatribe then there's nothing wrong with sampling a bit of the old "blue material" to see how everyone else does it. You can find everything you need from PG-13 rated movies and TV shows talking about sexy feelings and passionate love making...to a little more outrageous imagination by way of porn and erotica.

Lessons We Learn From Porn

Most people think of dirty talking as pornographic and not erotic. That's because porn has been dirty-talking for ages, while mainstream "classy erotica" is just now realizing that you can say "fuck" and not to have to clean it up for sensitive audiences. We're just not THAT sensitive anymore.

However, porn is not the "ideal" because it tends to be male-centric and over-the-top in terms of fantasy and bad acting. It also has a number of fetishes that may or may not be allowed in your bedroom like anal sex, cumshots to the face, cum swallowing and spitting and lesbian gangbangs.

If you and your partner are okay being a little wild, then it might work for you. But even if porn doesn't quite do it for you, there are some great lessons to learn. Such as:

Exaggerate your orgasmic intensity and arousal and it WILL feel better.

Dirty Talk #117: "Oh it's too much! Please stop! You're fucking me so good...I can't keep cumming all night! I'm going to faint!"

(Assuming your partner knows you're exaggerating, this can be a hot thing to say that's not exactly realistic, but still fun)

It's okay to objectify your partner's body.

Dirty Talk #118: "Take off your underwear. Let me see it. Now bend over. I want to see

all of you. I want to see you touch yourself for my amusement."

(Love and sex don't have to be the exact same thing. It's okay to treat your partner like an "object" since this is just a game and you're not bringing it outside the bedroom)

You don't have to be grounded in reality. It's OK to indulge your partner's naughty taboos sometimes.

Dirty Talk #119: "I'm going to ride your cock hard, while my sexy college roommate rubs my clit. Is this what you like, baby? Two girls fucking each other right on top of you?"

Porn isn't realistic but dirty talking doesn't have to be ultra-real. It just has to be sexual and sometimes a "quickie" short story about random fucking will do just fine.

Lessons We Learn From Erotica

Erotica has always had the literate angle, as sexual content that appeals to the mind. We can be thankful that erotica has given us the gift of plot, pace and timing, whereas porn has never been so concerned with effective moods or characterization. From erotica we get the psychological intensity and the slowly rising trepidation that turns into forbidden lust slowly but surely. It starts with a mood and then lights a fire that must be extinguished at all cost.

Dirty Talk #120: "You feel a flutter in your stomach. You know it's wrong. But my hand on your tummy is firm, and you know that I'm not going anywhere. I'm tired of resisting you. I can't live without you...your scent is driving me crazy. I just want to caress you, massage you, and make love to you. Right here. Right now. I can't wait till we go back to the room. I need you now. I slowly reach in and drop your panties to the floor..."

It is also thanks to erotica that we have the ability to "lose ourselves" and go well beyond our ordinary moral / ethical behavior, just so we can entertain some red-hot fantasies involving group sex, infidelity, and BDSM master-slave kink. We don't even have to "act". We can just read a story, or tell our own story with fictional characters. The erotic novel has given us permission to live vicariously through other people that have flaming libidos much more perverted than our own. Let's enjoy it.

Dirty Talk #121: "You've always been curious about how it would feel to have two men making love to you at the same time. Well, now it's your lucky day because I've taken in a sexy drifter and he thinks you're gorgeous. Maybe we should all have a few drinks and you can dance for us..."

Lessons We Learn from Phone Sex

Phone sex was big business back in the 1980s and 1990s, even though it's slowed down somewhat thanks to free Internet porn. But the interactive talk and non-visual element has affected our culture and our ability to experience intrigue, arousal and climax even without the necessity of a physical encounter.

Phone sex is all about firing up your imagination and using your hearing and speaking ability to create strong mental images that are just as good as porn but far more intense because YOU'RE the star of the show. Couples can take heed from this and keep their sex life booming even when separated by miles or in some cases, in a completely different time zone.

Phone sex gave us great visualizing dialog that still work today. With suggestions and sexual fantasy fulfillment we learned great lines like these:

Dirty Talk #122: "What are you wearing? What color are your panties? Are you sleeping in the nude? Are you touching yourself right now?"

Dirty Talk #123: "You want to cum together? Let's stroke at the same time and think of each other..."

Dirty Talk #124: "Tell your fantasy. Tell me all the dirty things you do when you jack off. I want to hear what a nasty little boy you are."

Lessons We Learn from Cyber Sex

The main difference between cyber sex and phone sex may well have been that in the old day, people that had phone sex NEVER intended on meeting in person. It was an erotic fantasy, with no intention of the two anonymous lovers ever meeting each other for a physical encounter. The cyber sex session, on the hand, thrives off the idea of actually meeting in person some day and getting to experience all of these fantasies in person. People often use the Internet for serious dating and so make Internet sex a mainstay in their virtual relationship.

This can continue onwards, even after you meet in person, and sometimes couples continue to have virtual sex even after marriage when they're separated on business or family travel. There is a sense of intimacy in cyber sex that is lacking in the business model of phone sex.

Therefore, cyber sex is all about the expectation, the emotion and feeling of what you want to do to and with your partner when you meet in person. This teaches us the thrill of preparing our partner, and building anticipation through phrases and explicit visuals. Such as:

Dirty Talk #125: "When we finally meet I just want to make sweet love to you for hours on end. I could spend all day between your legs just nibbling at your gorgeous body."

Dirty Talk #126: I want to place a 100 kisses all over you, from head to toe. I'm tired of waiting. I just want to reach out and take you into my arms...to be naked with you in bed, in the pool, in the kitchen, everywhere!"

Rather than phone sex, which works because of high emotion, multiple changes in voice tone, and the ability to hear each other's voice, text cyber sex works best in describing what we are FEELING, in the PRESENT. You don't just share fantasies or masturbate together, but actually tell your lover exactly how to feel with your simulated actions. As in:

Dirty Talk #127: "I'm touching your breasts right now...can you feel how my hands linger there, in awe of you, teasing your nipples until they're nice and puffy."

Dirty Talk #128: "You give me a wet and vicious hand job. And I love it. I tell you to do your worst. You stroke me, spit on me, and suck me and roughhouse me to your heart's desire. I want to lose control of myself, all in your hands..."

Dirty Talk #129: I enter the room and shove you down on the bed, feasting away at that beautiful bubbly ass of yours. I kiss it, deflowering your innocent flesh. I pull your ass cheeks apart getting a good look at your pussy and asshole. I stick my face right in your pussy lips, drunk on the taste of you, wanting to go deeper. I ask you to spread your legs and you obey, just as eager to surrender to me, as I am eager to conquer you."

True, by the time the web cam came along, Internet sex combined the best of three technologies: phone sex, text sex and even visual sex, thanks to high resolution displays that let lovers see each other in real time.

However, by the time the cell phone and tablet PC revolutionized chat, we were in for another social phenomenon: texting, or shall we say, SEXTING. This went one step beyond cyber sex, and was exclusively focused on building anticipation—in many cases, keeping your lover simmering on sexual thoughts for hours while at work.

That's the focus of the next chapter.

Chapter 13: How to Give Him or Her the Best "Sexting" Ever (Phrase 130-155)

It's just not that easy to go into explicit detail when sexting your partner with a mobile phone, including those awful virtual keyboards that are nearly impossible to type with...not to mention the difficulty in sexting with one hand!

Yes, it's fairly obvious that sexting is not the same thing as cyber sex or phone sex, since the time and place for intimacy is impractical. However, sexting is all about sharing THOUGHTS rather than full experiences. Another way to increase your partner's anticipation for sex later on, keeping them in a perpetual state of horny desire.

Of course, there are rules to sexting, and the most important ones are just a matter of decency and respect, since your partner will likely be rummaging through these text messages at work. It is advisable to not show your face if you're sending a nude picture and not to creep a new potential date out by "sexting" before you've had a chance to get intimate in person or on the phone. It's also not polite to keep your partner waiting for hours just for one reply, nor is it polite to send more than a few texts a day. (After all, your hot and bothered spouse still has to work!)

That said, sexting is a great tool to keep your partner's imagination fired up throughout long hours of all work and no play. Usually the best sext messages are very coy and teasing. They're not actually about having sex with words, but making your partner crave real sex later on with teases like:

Dirty Talk #130: "I just got you something very naughty. I think you're going to flip the fuck out when you see me in it tonight... ◉ "

Dirty Talk #131: "Oh God I can't stop thinking about you and last night. I can feel you on my hands, I can smell you all over. I need you now!"

Dirty Talk #132: "Just sitting here fantasizing about you...wondering how we could get in here afterhours and fuck on the desk."

Dirty Talk #133: "I want to have multiples with you."

Dirty Talk #134: I thought about you today...in the shower. ;)

In all of these examples, you notice the texting doesn't really go into great detail, as with the fantasy sharing dirty talking we discussed earlier. Just the implication that something mind blowing is going to happen is enough to fire him/her up.

In fact, you can get away with saying things on texting that are probably hard to say face to face without laughing. You can say cheesy sexual one liners like:

Dirty Talk #135: "I need a massage. But not so much a full body massage. Just your hands working their magic."

Dirty Talk #136: "I don't need porn. I just keep thinking of you in the nude and touching myself. God, I'm supposed to be working!"

Dirty Talk #137: "If you knew the naughty stuff I really think about you...you couldn't even look me in the eye!"

Dirty Talk #138: "I want a sundae...and I want to eat it off your body."

Dirty Talk #139: "Nice tie in that picture. But I thought of a much better use for it."

Another possibility is to use sexting as a means of making plans, or more specifically, playing dominant and submissive. You could do vanilla style commands like:

Dirty Talk #140: "I want to take you to a hotel room, tie you up, and make you scream. But no one will hear you. I'm going to cock tease you for hours."

Dirty Talk #141: "Tell me the color of your panties."

Dirty Talk #142: "I want a cock pic. NOW."

Dirty Talk #143: "Shock me with your sickest fantasy ever."

Dirty Talk #144: "You will be my toy tonight."

Dirty Talk #145: "Tell me the dirtiest thing you've ever thought about me."

Dirty Talk #146: "I'm just thinking about what a wet mess we're both going to be tomorrow morning..."

Or you could escalate the teasing into a full game of truth or dare with bold suggestions like:

Dirty Talk #147: "Text me a picture of your cleavage. I need my fix. Your body keeps my going."

Dirty Talk #148: "Go into the bathroom next break and masturbate. I will if you will."

Dirty Talk #149: "I have a JOB to give you...if you know what I mean. Interested in the POSITION?"

Dirty Talk #150: "Wear something with easy access tonight. I've waited long enough for a good fuck in public."

Dirty Talk #151: "I want to be used by you."

All in all, sexting is about embracing the fantasy, which will make the reality later that night so much hotter than a regular roll in the hay. You can push the limits of good taste in sexting because it's all a game. It's all flattery and X-rated compliments. You don't even have to put as much thought into a good sext as you might a full phone conversation.

Naked sexual desire shines through here. Sure, you're joking. You're being over the top and you're sometimes silly. But all you're really saying is that you desire your partner. You're so hot and bothered that you can't even go a whole day or day and a half without sending your wonderfully invasive sex fantasies.

You can even enhance your sex texts with semi-nude pictures, with sex toy pictures or kinky captions, or simply remark about your partner's photo and say something wildly inappropriate and NSFW.

Try:

Dirty Talk #152: "I like this vibrator. But I don't think it's powerful enough to compete with my tongue."

Dirty Talk #153: "Look how cute you look in this picture! Oops...I stared so long at your cute ass I have to change my clothes now."

Dirty Talk #154: "Up skirt picture for you. Just reminding you of where you're going tonight."

Dirty Talk #155: "Now I'm just sending you random pictures of landmarks I want to fuck you in..."

Thankfully, only you have the password to your cellphone so all of this is locked away for good. In short, this is legal and ethical sexual harassment. Have some fun with it. In fact, you should try to push the boundaries just a little bit and see how horny you can make your partner with badboy/badgirl texts.

Don't respect your partner so much that you're afraid to be silly, or immature or even a little selfish and crude. In fact, the more ill-behaved you are in sexting, the more your partner seems to crave it. It gives each of you something nice and kinky to look forward to in between calls, tasks and lunch breaks.

Yes, sexting is a wonderful treat, something that reminds us how much fun courtship and dating can be...even if you've been married for eons!

Speaking of which, it's time to discuss some other great avenues for dirty talking that you might not have considered yet. It is an art that can be used in practically every situation you might encounter in this roller coaster ride we call life. Let's proceed into Chapter 14.

Chapter 14: Dirty Talking for Every Situation in Life (Phrase 156-157)

What's nice about dirty talking, as a regular part of your ongoing sex life, is that it is flexible to whatever living situation you have. Couples use dirty talking in all aspects of their active lives including:

- Sexting at work

- Spicing up their sexual foreplay with dialog

- Using dirty talking during sex, to heighten orgasm

- Enjoying quickies with toys and a shared fantasy

- Enjoying intimacy while away from each other, through web cam, phone or texting

- Helping to boost each other's confidence

- Improving creativity and keeping sex spontaneous

- Resisting outside temptations since dirty talking and fantasies address these needs and desires

- Boosting your lover's self-esteem with a funny or sexy text when he or she is feeling down.

- Improving communication and your overall relationship

Yes, relationships are built on good communication and stay strong through constant reinforcement of intimacy. Dirty talking can help in this regard because it constantly challenges you, keeping you on your feet, reminding you of how young and rebellious we all can be at any moment in time.

This is solid communication and game-playing that can stand the test of time, keeping lovers red hot and interested in each other from now and into their golden years. It doesn't even matter if looks fade or if life situations change. Your minds will always be connected, always in love, and always full of passion for each other.

Dirty Talk #156: "You're as drop dead sexy now as you were when I first met you. Every day my desire for you grows stronger. You're an addiction of mine that grows. Every passing day I crave more of you, want all of you and it's never enough."

Dirty Talk #157: "Are you still mad at me? Just because I am a constantly running sex machine doesn't mean I'm not a romantic. You're the most beautiful person in the world and I will always love you uncontrollably."

Bonus #1: "Whatever happens for the rest of our lives...just remember...I nailed you. I banged you good and you liked it. Happy anniversary, lover!"

Dirty Talk is Not Just Foreplay – It's Honest to Goodness Sex!

Don't think that dirty talk is just one more way of saying "foreplay." While it can be used effectively in foreplay, it is an honest-to-goodness sexual technique, just as valid as intercourse, oral sex and mutual masturbation. It is a form of intimacy and sexual behavior, and many lovers are completely satisfied to just have sexting or fantasy sharing than they are actual intercourse. Sometimes our imagination is all that needs to be stimulated.

Some men and woman suffering from disabilities, such as paralysis or paraplegia, take joy in dirty talking, as it's a form of sexual stimulation that doesn't require physical exertion. People who cannot enjoy sex due to illness or age-related condition can still enjoy eroticism and romance, by exercising their brains and using their wild imaginations in brand new scenarios.

Bonus #2: "Would you fuck me in a car? Would you lick me in a bar? Would you ride me on a boat? Would you screw me on a float? Would you bang me on a plane? Would you spank me with a cane? Would

you make love to me in rhyme? Would you do me until the end of time?"

Bonus #3: "Tell me your deepest and most hidden thoughts. Nothing you could ever say would shock me. In fact, I'd probably say, 'Let's try it once."

Besides, did you know that orgasm is an entirely mental process? We all think of it as a physical response. And while it is brought on by stimulation, many people can actually "think" their way to orgasm by entertaining sexual fantasies and focusing on their erotic sensations. Dirty talking, with its limitless possibilities and no-holds-barred approach to honest communication, is certainly a way to help enhance orgasm—in the bedroom and out.

Conclusion

I hope you've enjoyed reading this book.

Sex is indeed a driving force in life. Romance and communication with our soul mate is one of the very few absolutes in the world. It's nothing to take for granted and it's something far too precious to let slip away.

Don't suppress your instincts. Sharpen them. Embrace possibility rather than fighting change. By having a bit of naughty fun you can help to keep your loving relationship strong, now and forever.

Made in the USA
Columbia, SC
30 November 2022